Taking Time

SUPPORT FOR PEOPLE WITH CANCER AND THE PEOPLE WHO CARE ABOUT THEM

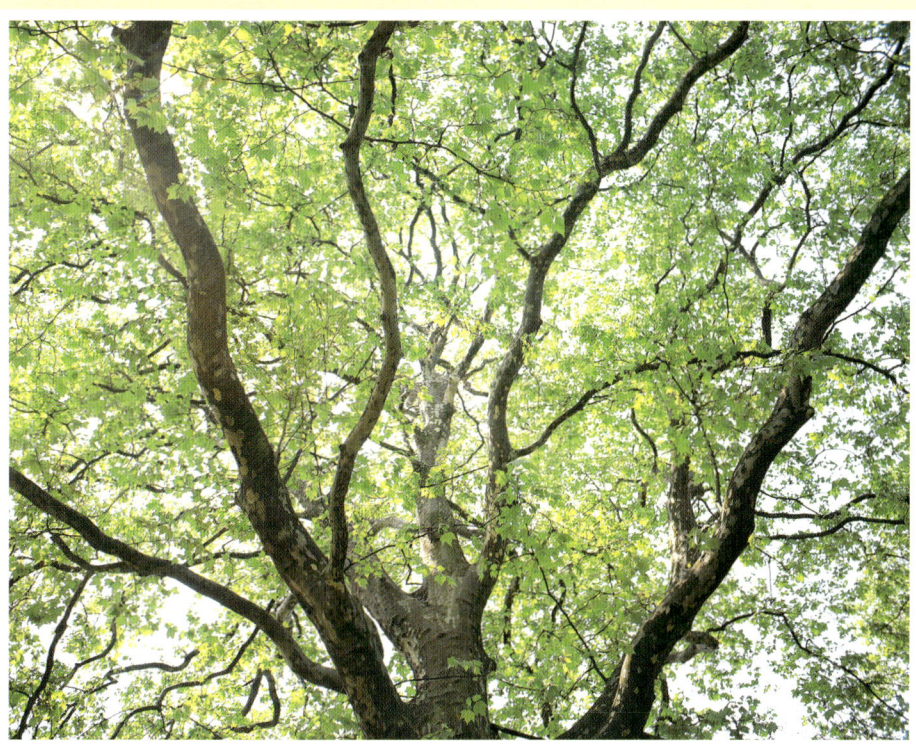

Living with cancer is hard. Where are you in this challenge?
You may have just learned that you have cancer. Or you may be
in treatment. At every point, you may have a range of feelings.
It is important to accept these feelings and learn how to live with them.
Feelings about your cancer may be with you for a long time.

This book was written for you—the person with cancer.
But this book can also be helpful to those people who are close to you.
This book may help them better understand what you are going through.
Even if you have no close relatives or live far away from your family,
you may have friends who you think of as your "family."
Whatever "family" means to you, share this book
with those who love and care about you.

Table of Contents

Introduction iv
    How to Use This Book v

1. Your Feelings: Learning You Have Cancer 1
    Denial 2
    Anger 3
    Fear and Worry 3
    Stress 4
    Pain 5
    Control and Self-Esteem 7
    Sadness and Depression 8
    Guilt 9
    Loneliness 9
    Hope 10
    Summing Up: Learning You Have Cancer 11

2. Family Matters 13
    Changes to Your Roles in the Family 14
    Spouses and Partners 16
    Children 17
    Adult Children 20
    Parents 22
    Close Friends 22
    Summing Up: Cancer and Your Family 23

3. Sharing Your Feelings About Cancer 25
    Friends and Family Have Feelings About Your Cancer 25
    Finding a Good Listener 26
    Choosing a Good Time to Talk 26
    Expressing Anger 27
    Pretending to Be Cheerful 28

Sharing Without Talking 28

Summing Up: Sharing Your Thoughts and Feelings About Cancer.....29

4. Learning About Your Cancer and Feeling More in Control..................31

Learning From Your Health Care Providers...32

Learning About Your Treatment Choices 33

Learning More About Your Cancer 34

Summing Up: Learning About Your Cancer and Regaining Control......35

5. People Helping People...37

Family and Friends..38

Other People Who Have Cancer 38

Support Groups...39

Spiritual Help..41

People in Health Care 42

People in the Hospital...45

Caregivers 46

Summing Up: People Helping People...49

6. Dealing with a New Self-Image..51

Fatigue 52

Your Self-Image 52

Staying Active 53

Getting Help..53

Facing Cancer with Your Spouse or Partner 54

Dating 55

Summing Up: Dealing with a New Self-Image.......................................56

7. Living Each Day 58

Keeping Up With Your Daily Routine 58

Working 60

Thinking About the Future 62

Summing Up: Living Each Day...64

Resources for Learning More 65

Introduction

Cancer Will Change Your Life

Cancer is a major illness, but not everyone who gets cancer will die from it. Close to 9 million Americans alive today have a history of cancer. For them, cancer has become a chronic (on-going) health problem, like high blood pressure or diabetes.

Just like anyone with a chronic health problem, people who have cancer must get regular checkups for the rest of their lives, even after cancer treatment ends. But unlike other chronic health problems, if you have cancer you probably will not need to take medicine or eat special foods once you have finished treatment.

If you have cancer, you may notice every ache, pain, or sign of illness. Even little aches may make you worry. While it is normal to think about dying and healthy to explore your feelings about death, it is also important to focus on living. Keep in mind that cancer is not a death sentence. Many people with cancer are treated successfully. Others will live a long time before dying from cancer. So, make the most of each day while living with cancer and its treatment.

> No one knows the story of tomorrow's dawn.
> —*Ashanti (African) Proverb*

People Respond to Cancer in Many Ways

This book was written to help you learn from other people with cancer. Finding out how others respond to cancer might help you understand your own feelings. Learning how others manage the special problems that cancer brings might help you find your own ways of coping with the problems that come along for you.

Sharing Ideas about Ways to Live with Cancer

Many people helped to write this book—people who have had cancer and their family members, friends, and caregivers. We thank each of them for sharing their ideas and suggestions about ways to live with cancer. You will find their comments in italic type throughout this book.

We also thank the many health care providers who reviewed *Taking Time*. Their comments and practical suggestions are based on years of experience helping people with cancer.

How to Use This Book

No two people are alike. Some chapters of this book may apply to your situation and others may not. Read the chapters that have meaning to you. The other chapters may be useful later on.

This book is divided into 7 chapters, plus a resource section at the end. Use the Table of Contents to find the section of the book that's most important to you during your treatment. Each chapter begins with a "Read This First" box, which tells you what is in that chapter. In addition, each chapter ends with a "Summing Up" box, which repeats the key ideas in that chapter.

As you read this booklet, remember, right now—it's all about you!

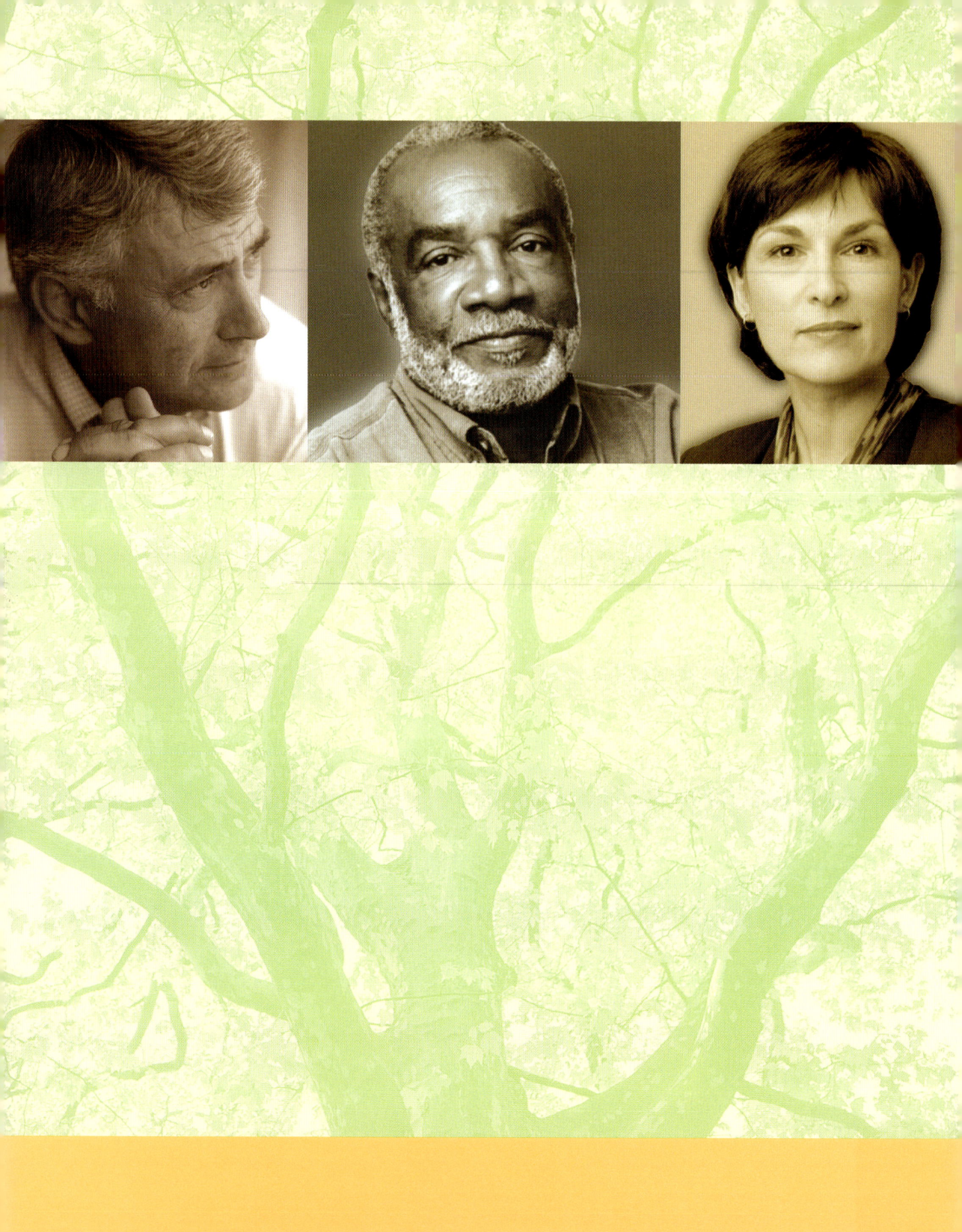

CHAPTER 1

Your Feelings: Learning You Have Cancer

You will have many feelings after you learn that you have cancer. These feelings can change from day to day, hour to hour, or even minute to minute.

Some of the feelings you may go through include:

- denial
- anger
- fear
- stress
- anxiety
- depression
- sadness
- guilt
- loneliness

All these feelings are normal.

Feeling hopeful is also normal. No one is cheerful all the time, but while you are dealing with cancer, hope can be an important part of your life.

"I heard the doctor say, 'I'm sorry; the test results show that you have cancer.' I heard nothing else. My mind went blank, and then I kept thinking, 'No, there must be some mistake.'"

Learning that you have cancer can come as a shock. How did you react? You may have felt numb, frightened, or angry. You may not have believed what the doctor was saying. You may have felt all alone, even if your friends and family were in the same room with you. These feelings are all normal.

For many people, the first few weeks after diagnosis are very difficult. After you hear the word "cancer," you may have trouble breathing or listening to what is being said. When you are at home, you may have trouble thinking, eating, or sleeping.

People with cancer and those close to them experience a wide range of feelings and emotions. These feelings can change often and without warning.

At times, you may:

- be angry, afraid, or worried
- not really believe that you have cancer
- feel out of control and not able to care for yourself
- be sad, guilty, or lonely
- have a strong sense of hope for the future

This chapter looks at many of the feelings that come up when people find out they have cancer.

Denial

When you were first diagnosed, you may have had trouble believing or accepting the fact that you have cancer. This is called denial. Denial can be helpful because it can give you time to adjust to your diagnosis. Denial can also give you time to feel hopeful and better about the future.

Sometimes, denial is a serious problem. If it lasts too long, it can keep you from getting the treatment you need. It can also be a problem when other people deny that you have cancer, even after you have accepted it.

The good news is that most people (those with cancer as well as those they love and care about) work through denial. By the time treatment begins, most people accept the fact that they have cancer.

Anger

Once you accept that you have cancer, you may feel angry and scared. It is normal to ask "Why me?" and be angry at:

- the cancer
- your health care providers
- your healthy friends and loved ones

And if you are religious, you might even be angry with God.

Anger sometimes comes from feelings that are hard to show—such as fear, panic, frustration, anxiety, or helplessness. If you feel angry, don't pretend that everything is okay. Talk with your family and friends about your anger. Most of the time, talking will help you feel a lot better. (See Chapter 3, "Sharing Your Feelings About Cancer.")

> Talking to one another is loving one another.
> —*Kenyan Proverb*

Fear and Worry

"The word 'cancer' frightens everyone I know. It's a diagnosis that most people fear more than any other."

It's scary to hear that you have cancer. You may be afraid or worried about:

- being in pain, either from the cancer or the treatment
- feeling sick or looking different as a result of your treatment
- taking care of your family
- paying your bills
- keeping your job
- dying

Your family and close friends may also worry about:

- seeing you upset or in pain
- not giving you enough support, love, and understanding
- living without you

Some fears about cancer are based on stories, rumors, and old information. Most people feel better when they know what to expect. They feel less afraid when they learn about cancer and its treatment. As one man with prostate cancer said,

"I read as much as I can find about my cancer. Imagining the worst is more frightening than knowing what might happen. Knowing the facts makes me much less afraid."

Stress

Your body may react to the stress and worry of having cancer. You may notice that:

- your heart beats faster
- you have headaches or muscle pains
- you don't feel like eating
- you feel sick to your stomach or have diarrhea
- you feel shaky, weak, or dizzy
- you have a tight feeling in your throat and chest
- you sleep too much or too little

Stress can also keep your body from fighting disease as well as it should.

You can learn to handle stress in many ways, like:

- exercising
- listening to music

- reading books, poems, or magazines
- getting involved in hobbies such as music or crafts
- relaxing or meditating, such as lying down and slowly breathing in and out
- talking about your feelings with family and close friends

If you are concerned about stress, talk to your doctor or nurse. He or she may be able to help you by referring you to a counselor or support group. You may also join a class that teaches people ways of dealing with stress. The key is to find ways to control stress and not to let it control you.

Pain

Even though almost everyone worries about pain, it may not be a problem for you. Some people do not have any pain. Others have pain only once in a while. Cancer pain can almost always be relieved. If you are in pain, your doctor can suggest ways to help you feel better. These include:

- prescription or over-the-counter medicines
- cold packs or heating pads
- relaxation, like getting a massage or listening to soothing music
- imagery, such as thinking about a place where you feel happy and calm
- distraction, like watching a movie, working on a hobby, or anything that helps take your mind off your pain

There is no reason for you to be bothered with pain. There are many ways to control pain. Your doctor wants and needs to hear about your pain. As soon as you have pain you should speak up. Dealing with your pain can also help you deal with the feelings discussed in this chapter.

> If you conceal your disease, you cannot expect to be cured.
> —*Ethiopian Proverb*

Pain Scales and Pain Journals

Pain scales or pain journals are tools that you can use to describe how much pain you feel. These tools can also help your doctor, nurse, or pharmacist find ways to treat your pain.

You are the only person who can decide how much pain you feel. When it comes to pain, there is no right or wrong answer. On many pain scales, you are asked to rate your pain as a number from 0 to 10. For example, you would rate your pain as "0" if you feel no pain at all. You would rate your pain as "10" if it is the worst pain you have ever felt in your life. You can pick any number between 0 and 10 to describe your pain.

When you use a pain scale, be sure to include the range. For example, you might say, "Today my pain is a 7 on a scale from 0 to 10."

A pain journal or diary is another tool you can use to describe your pain. With a journal or diary, you not only use a pain scale but also write down what you think causes your pain and what helps you feel better.

When you describe your pain to your doctor, nurse, pharmacist, or family member, tell them:

- where you feel pain
- what it feels like (sharp, dull, throbbing, steady)
- how strong the pain feels
- how long it lasts
- what eases the pain and what makes it worse
- what medicines you are taking for the pain and how much they help

To find out more about pain, contact the Cancer Information Service or look online at **http://cancer.gov** (see "Resources for Learning More" on page 65).

Control and Self-Esteem

When you first learn that you have cancer, you may feel as if your life is out of control. You may feel this way because:

- you wonder if you will live or die
- your daily routine is messed up by doctor visits and treatments
- people use medical words and terms that you don't understand
- you feel like you can't do things you enjoy
- you feel helpless
- the health professionals treating you are strangers

Even though you may feel out of control, there are ways you can be in charge. For example, you can:

- **Learn as much as you can about your cancer.** You can call 1-800-4-CANCER (1-800-422-6237) or TTY (for deaf and hard of hearing callers) at 1-800-332-8615. You can also go online at http://cancer.gov and click on "LiveHelp" at the lower right. (See Chapter 4, "Learning About Your Cancer and Feeling More in Control.")

- **Ask questions.** Let your health providers know when you don't understand what they are saying, or when you want more information about something.

- **Look beyond your cancer.** Many people with cancer feel better when they stay busy. You may still go to work, even if you need to adjust your schedule. You can also take part in hobbies such as music, crafts, or reading.

As one woman with cancer commented,

"Once I started to feel better, I found myself looking for new outlets for creativity. I had always promised myself that some day I would take a photography course. My satisfaction with my new hobby helped me feel better about other areas of my life as well."

Sadness and Depression

Many people with cancer feel sad or depressed. This is a normal response to any serious illness. When you're depressed, you may have very little energy, feel tired, or not want to eat.

Depression is sometimes a serious problem. If feelings of sadness and despair seem to take over your life, you may have clinical depression. The box below lists eight common signs of depression. Let your health provider know if you have one or more of these signs almost every day.

Early Signs of Depression

Check the signs that are problems for you:

- a feeling that you are helpless and hopeless, or that life has no meaning
- no interest in being with your family or friends
- no interest in the hobbies and activities you used to enjoy
- a loss of appetite, or no interest in food
- crying for long periods of time, or many times each day
- sleep problems, either sleeping too much or too little
- changes in your energy level
- thoughts of killing yourself. This includes making plans or taking action to kill yourself, as well as frequent thoughts about death and dying.

Depression can be treated. Your doctor may prescribe medication. He or she may also suggest that you talk about your feelings with a counselor or join a support group with others who have cancer.

> Turn your face to the sun and the shadows fall behind you.
> —*Maori Proverb*

Guilt

Many people with cancer feel guilty. For example, you may blame yourself for upsetting the people you love. You may worry that you are a burden to others, either emotionally or financially. Or you may envy other people's good health and be ashamed of this feeling. You might even blame yourself for lifestyle choices that could have led to your cancer. For example, that lying out in the sun caused your skin cancer or that smoking cigarettes led to your lung cancer.

These feelings are all normal for people with cancer. One woman with breast cancer said,

"When I feel guilty that I caused my cancer, I think of little children who have cancer. That makes me realize that cancer can just happen. It isn't my fault."

Your family and friends may also feel guilty because:

- they are healthy while you are ill
- they can't help you as much as they want
- they feel stressed and impatient

They may also want to be perfect and feel guilty when they cannot give you all the care and understanding you need.

Counseling and support groups can help with these feelings of guilt. Let your doctor or nurse know if you, or someone in your family, would like to talk with a counselor or go to a support group.

Loneliness

People with cancer often feel lonely or distant from others. You may find that your friends have a hard time dealing with your cancer and may not visit. Some people might not even be able to call you on the phone. You may feel too sick to take part in the hobbies and activities you used to enjoy. And sometimes, even when you are with people you love and care about, you may feel that no one understands what you are going through.

You may feel less lonely when you meet other people who have cancer. Many people feel better when they join a support group and talk with others who are facing the same challenges. (See Chapter 5, "People Helping People.")

> Shared joy is a double joy; shared sorrow is half a sorrow.
> —*Swedish Proverb*

Not everyone wants or is able to join a support group. Some people prefer to talk with just one person at a time. You may feel better talking to a close friend or family member, someone from your own religion, or a counselor.

Hope

Once people accept that they have cancer, they often feel a sense of hope. There are many reasons to feel hopeful.

- Cancer treatment can be successful. Millions of people who have had cancer are alive today.
- People with cancer can lead active lives, even during treatment.
- Your chances of living with—and living beyond—cancer are better now than they have ever been before. People often live for many years after their cancer treatment is over.

Some doctors think that hope may help your body deal with cancer. Scientists are looking at the question of whether a hopeful outlook and positive attitude helps people feel better. Here are some ways you can build your sense of hope:

- Write down your hopeful feelings and talk about them with others.
- Plan your days as you always have done.
- Don't limit the things you like to do just because you have cancer.
- Look for reasons to hope.

> However long the night, the dawn will break.
> —*Hausa (African) Proverb*

You may find hope in nature, or your religious or spiritual beliefs. Or you may find hope in stories (such as the ones in this book) about people with cancer who are leading active lives.

Summing Up: Learning You Have Cancer

You will have many feelings as you learn to live with cancer. These feelings can change from day to day, hour to hour, or even minute to minute.

Feelings of denial, anger, fear, stress and anxiety, depression, sadness, guilt, and loneliness are all normal. So is a feeling of hope. While no one is cheerful all the time, hope is a normal and positive part of your cancer experience.

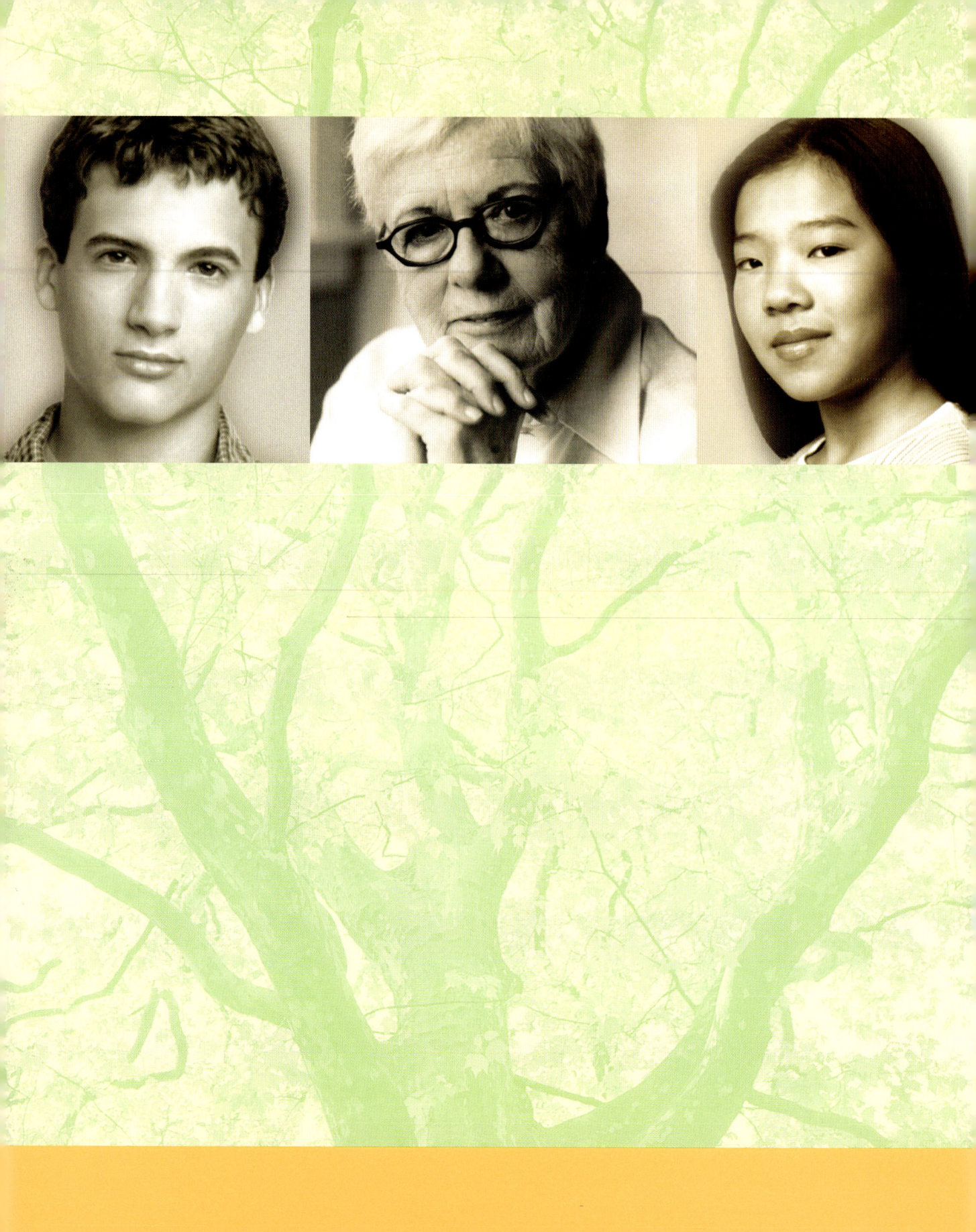

CHAPTER 2

Family Matters

Cancer will change your life and the lives of people around you.

- Your routines may be messed up.
- Roles and duties may change.
- Relationships can be strained or strengthened.
- Dealing with money and insurance can cause problems.
- You may need to live with someone else for a while.
- You may need help with chores and errands.

Most people find that if they, their friends, and family talk about the cancer and how it makes them feel, they feel closer to each other.

Families are not all alike. Your family may include a spouse (husband or wife), children, and parents. Or maybe you think of your partner or close friends as your family. In this book, "family" refers to you and those who love and support you.

Cancer affects the whole family, not just the person with the disease. How are the people in your family dealing with your cancer? Maybe they are afraid or angry, just like you.

When you first find out you have cancer and are going through treatments, day-to-day routines may change for everyone. For example, someone in your family may need to take time off work to drive you to treatments. You may need help with chores and errands.

How your family reacts to your cancer may depend a lot on how you've faced hard times in the past.

Some families find it easy to talk about cancer. They may easily share their feelings about the changes that cancer brings to their lives. Other families find it harder to talk about cancer. The people in these families may be used to solving problems alone and not want to talk about their feelings.

Families that have gone through divorce or had other losses may have even more trouble talking about cancer. As one woman with lung cancer said,

"Talking about my cancer was rough at first. My husband and I divorced five years ago, so my mom had to move in and help me with the boys. Eventually, I was able to tell my ex-husband about my cancer, and he helped the boys understand. Our family has been through a lot, and we'll get through this, too. To me, the only constant in life is change."

If your family is having trouble talking about feelings, think about getting some help. Your doctor or nurse can refer you to a counselor who can help people in your family talk about what cancer means to them. Many families find that, even though it can be hard to do, they feel close to each other when they deal with cancer together.

Changes to Your Roles in the Family

When someone in a family has cancer, everyone takes on new roles and responsibilities. For example, a child may be asked to do more chores or a spouse or partner may need to help pay bills, shop, or do yard work. Family members sometimes have trouble adjusting to these new roles.

Adjusting to Your New Situation

Many families have trouble getting used to the role changes that may be required when a loved one has cancer.

Money. Cancer can reduce the amount of money your family has to spend or save. If you are not able to work, someone else in your family may need to get a job. You and your family will need to learn more about health insurance and find out what your insurance will pay for and what you need to pay for. Most people find it stressful to keep up with money matters. (For more information about cancer and your work, see Chapter 7, "Living Each Day" on page 57.)

Living arrangements. People with cancer sometimes need to change where they live or whom they live with. Now that you have cancer, you may need to move in with someone else to get the care you need. This can be hard because you may feel that you are losing your independence, at least for a little while. Or, you may need to travel far from home for treatment. If you have to be away from home for treatments take a few little things from home with you. This way, there will be something familiar even in a strange place.

Daily activities. You may need help with duties such as paying bills, cooking meals, or coaching your children's teams. Asking others to do these things for you can be hard. A young father in treatment for colon cancer said,

"When I came home from the hospital, I wanted to be in charge again but simply didn't have the energy. It was so hard to ask for help! It was easier to accept help when I realized that my kids felt that they were contributing to my recovery."

Developing a Plan

Even when others offer to help, it is important to let people know that you can still do some things for yourself. As much as you are able, keep up with your normal routine by making decisions, doing household chores, and working on hobbies that you enjoy.

Asking for help is not a sign of weakness. Think about hiring someone or asking for a volunteer. Health insurance sometimes pays for people to help with household chores. You might be able to find a volunteer through groups in your community.

Paid help or volunteers may be able to help with:

- physical care, such as bathing or dressing
- household chores, such as cleaning or food shopping
- skilled care, such as giving you special feedings or medications

Just as you need time for yourself, your family members also need time to rest, have fun, and take care of their other duties. Respite care is a way people can get the time they need. In respite care, someone comes to your home and takes care of you while your family member goes out for a while. Let your doctor or social worker know if you want to learn more about respite care. (See Chapter 5, "People Helping People.")

Spouses and Partners

"I was scared by my husband's cancer. He had always taken care of me and we did everything together. I was afraid I would not be strong enough to help him through his recovery. I was afraid that he might not recover. I was afraid to talk about my fears with him because I did not want to upset him."

Your husband, wife, or partner may feel just as scared by cancer as you do. You both may feel anxious, helpless, or afraid. You may find it hard to be taken care of by someone you love.

People react to cancer in different ways. Some cannot accept that cancer is a serious illness. Others try too hard to be "perfect" caregivers. And some people refuse to talk about cancer. For most people, thinking about the future is scary.

It helps if you and the people close to you can talk about your fears and concerns. You may want to meet with a counselor who can help both of you talk about these feelings.

Sharing Information

Including your spouse or partner in treatment decisions is important. You can meet with your doctor together and learn about your type of cancer. You might want to find out about common symptoms, treatment choices, and their side effects. This information will help both of you plan for the future.

Your spouse or partner will also need to know how to help take care of your body and your feelings. And, even though it is not easy, both of you should think about the future and make plans in case you die from your cancer. You may find it helpful to meet with a financial planner or a lawyer.

Staying Close

Everyone needs to feel needed and loved. You may have always been the "strong one" in your family, but now is the time to let your spouse or partner help you. This can be as simple as letting the other person fluff your pillow, bring you a cool drink, or read to you.

Feeling sexually close to your partner is also important. You may not be interested in sex when you are in treatment because you feel tired, sick to your stomach, or in pain. But when your treatment is over, you may want to have sex again. Until then, you and your spouse or partner may need to find new ways to show that you care about each other. This can include touching, holding, hugging, and cuddling. (See also Chapter 6, "Dealing with a New Self-Image.")

Time Away

Your spouse or partner needs to keep a sense of balance in his or her life. He or she needs time to take care of personal chores and errands. Your partner will also need time to sort through his or her own feelings about cancer. And most importantly, everyone needs time to rest. If you do not want to be alone when your loved one is away, think about getting respite care or asking a friend to stay with you. (See "Caregivers" on page 46.)

Children

Even though your children will be sad and upset when they learn about your cancer, do not pretend that everything is okay. Even very young children can sense when something is wrong. They will see that you do not feel well or are not spending as much time with them as you used to. They may notice that you have a lot of visitors and phone calls or that you need to be away from home for treatment and doctor's visits.

> What the family talks about in the evening, the child will talk about in the morning.
> —Kenyan Proverb

Telling Children About Cancer

Children as young as 18 months old begin to think about and understand what is going on around them. It is important to be honest and tell your children that you are sick and the doctors are working to make you better. Telling them the truth is better than letting them imagine the worst. Give your children time to ask questions and express their feelings. And if they ask questions that you can't answer, let them know that you will find out the answers for them.

When you talk with your children, use words and terms they can understand. For example, say "doctor" instead of "oncologist" or "medicine" instead of "chemotherapy." Tell your children how much you love them and suggest ways they can help with your care. Share books about cancer that are written for children. Your doctor, nurse, or social worker can suggest good ones for your child.

Let other adults in your children's lives know about your cancer. This includes teachers, neighbors, coaches, or other relatives who can spend extra time with them. These other adults may be able to take your children to their activities, as well as listen to their feelings and concerns. Your doctor or nurse can also help by talking with your children and answering their questions.

How Children May React

Children can react to cancer in many different ways. For example, they may:

- be confused, scared, or lonely
- feel guilty and think that something they did or said caused your cancer
- feel angry when they are asked to be quiet or do more chores around the house
- miss the amount of attention they are used to getting
- regress and behave as they did when they were much younger
- get into trouble at school or at home
- be clingy and afraid to leave the house

"Now that my Mom has cancer, everything is changed. I want to be with her, but I want to hang out with my friends, too. She needs me to help with my little brother, but what I really want to do is play football like I used to."

Teenagers and a Parent's Cancer

Teens are at a time in their lives when they are trying to break away and be independent from their parents. When a parent has cancer, breaking away can be hard for them to do. They may become angry, act out, or get into trouble.

Try to get your teens to talk about their feelings. Tell them as much as they want to know about your cancer. Ask them for their opinions and, if possible, let them help you make decisions.

Teens may want to talk with other people in their lives. Friends can be a great source of support, especially those who also have serious illness in their family. Other family members, teachers, coaches, and spiritual leaders can also help. Encourage your teenage children to talk about their fears and feelings with people they trust and feel close to. Some towns even have support groups for teens whose parents have cancer.

What children of all ages need to know:

About cancer

- Nothing your child did, thought, or said caused you to get cancer.

- You can't catch cancer from another person. Just because you have cancer does not mean that others in your family will get it, too.

- Just because you have cancer does not mean you will die from it. In fact, many people live with cancer for a long time.

- Scientists are finding many new ways to treat cancer.

About living with cancer in the family

- Your child is not alone. Other children have parents who have cancer.

- It is okay to be upset, angry, or scared about your illness.

- Your child can't do anything to change the fact that you have cancer.

- Family members may act differently because they are worried about you.

- You will make sure that your children are taken care of, no matter what happens to you.

About what they can do

- They can help you by doing nice things like washing dishes or drawing you a picture.

- They should still go to school and take part in sports and other fun activities.

- They can talk to other adults such as teachers, family members, and religious leaders.

Adult Children

Your relationship with your adult children may change now that you have cancer. You may:

- Ask your adult children to take on new duties, such as making health care decisions, paying bills, or taking care of the house.

- Ask your children to explain some of the information you've received from your doctor or to go with you to doctor's visits so they can also hear what the doctors are telling you.

- Rely on your adult children for emotional support. For instance, you may ask them to act as "go-betweens" with friends or other family members.

- Want your adult children to spend a lot of time with you. This can be hard, especially if they have jobs or young families of their own.

- Find it hard to receive—rather than give—comfort and support from your children.

- Feel awkward when your children help with your physical care, such as feeding or bathing.

As the adult daughter of a woman with ovarian cancer said,

"Mom was always the rock in the family. Whenever any of us had a problem, we could go to her for help. Now we had to help her. It was almost as though we were the parents and she was the child. To make it even harder, we had our own children to take care of and jobs to go to."

Talking With Your Adult Children

It is important to talk about cancer with your adult children, even if they get upset or worry about you. Include them when talking about your treatment. Let them know your thoughts and wishes, in case you do not recover from your cancer.

Even adult children worry that their parents will die. When they learn that you have cancer, adult children may realize how important you are to them. They may feel guilty if they haven't been close with you. They may feel bad if they cannot spend a lot of time with you because they live far away or have other duties. Some of these feelings may make it harder to talk to your adult children. If you have trouble talking with your adult children, ask your doctor or nurse to suggest a counselor you can all talk with.

Make the most of the time you have with your adult children. Talk about how much you mean to each other. Express all your feelings—not just love but also anxiety, sadness, and anger. Don't worry about saying the wrong thing. It's better to share your feelings rather than hide them.

> One who conceals grief finds no remedy for it.
> —*Turkish Proverb*

Cancer Risk for the Children of People Who Have Cancer

Now that you have cancer, your children may wonder about their chance of getting it as well. Suggest they talk with a doctor about their risk of getting cancer.

A higher risk for some types of cancer are passed from parent to child. For instance, the daughter of a woman with breast cancer may be at risk for getting the same disease. But chances are that her risk is no different than other women her age. If concerned, however, children should talk with a doctor about their risk of getting cancer.

Gene tests can be a way to find out if a person is at higher risk of getting cancer. Although some gene tests can be helpful, they do not always give people the kinds of answers they are seeking. Talk to your doctor if you or someone in your family wants to learn more about gene testing for cancer. He or she can refer you to a person who is specially trained in this area. These experts can help you think through your choices and answer your questions.

Parents

Since people are living much longer these days, many people with cancer may also be caring for their aging parents. For example, you may help your parents with their shopping or take them to doctor. Your aging parents may even live with you.

You have to decide how much to tell your parents about your cancer. Your decision may depend on how well your parents can understand and cope with the news. If your parents are in good health, think about talking with them about your cancer.

Now that you have cancer, you may need extra help caring for your parents. You may need help only while you are in treatment. Or you may need to make long-term changes in your parents' care. Talk with your family members, friends, health professionals, and community agencies to see how they can help. (See Chapter 5, "People Helping People")

Close Friends

> Do not protect yourself by a fence, but rather by your friends.
> —*Czech Proverb*

Once friends learn of your cancer, they may begin to worry. Some will ask you to tell them ways to help. Others will wonder how they can help but may not know how to ask. You can help your friends cope with the news by letting them help you in some way. Think about the things your friends do well and don't mind doing. Make a list of things you think you might need. This way, when they ask you how they can be of help, you'll be able to share your list of needs and allow them to pick something they're willing to do.

Sample list of need:

- Baby-sit on days that I go to treatment.
- Prepare frozen meals for my "down days."
- Put my name on the prayer list at my place of worship.
- Bring me a few books from the library when you go.

- Visit for tea or coffee when you can.
- Let others know that it is alright to call or visit me (or let others know that I'm not ready for visitors just yet).

Summing Up: Cancer and Your Family

Families come in many forms. Some are husband, wife, and children. Others are life partners. Still others are groups of people who love and support each other.

No matter what form your family takes, your cancer will not only change your life, but also the lives of those around you.

Cancer impacts families in different ways.

- Talking about cancer can be hard for some families.
- Routines of family life may be messed up.
- Roles and duties within the family will change.
- Relationships can be both strained and strengthened.
- Dealing with money and insurance often become hard.
- You may need to change where you live and with whom, at least for a while.

As you think about how cancer has changed your life and your family's life, think about reaching outside your family to get help.

- You may need help with household chores and errands.
- Respite care can give your regular caregivers a much-needed break.
- Counseling and support groups can help your family deal with the issues that cancer raises.

Most families find that being honest and open about the cancer, about the problems that arise, and about their feelings, helps them handle the changes that cancer causes.

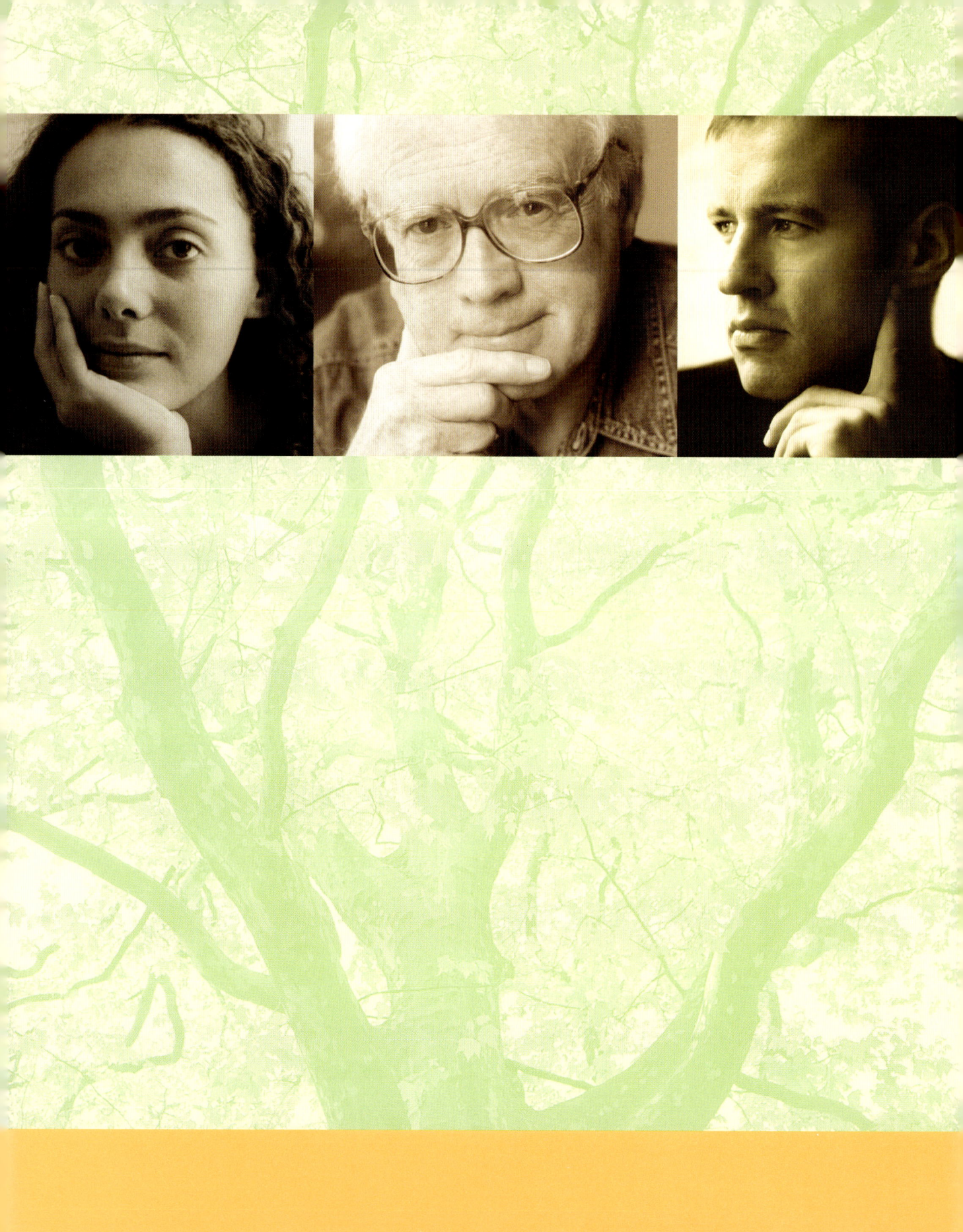

CHAPTER 3

Sharing Your Feelings About Cancer

Talking about your feelings can help you deal with your cancer.

- Choose a good listener.
- Choose a good time to share your feelings.
- Understand your feelings of anger.
- Don't act cheerful when you don't feel that way.

You may need to find someone outside your family to talk to.

Cancer is too much to handle all by yourself.

Your Friends and Family Have Feelings About Your Cancer

Just as you have strong feelings about cancer, your family or friends will react to it as well. For instance, your friends or family may:

- hide or deny their sad feelings
- find someone to blame for your cancer
- change the subject when someone talks about cancer
- act mad for no real reason
- make jokes about cancer
- pretend to be cheerful all the time
- avoid talking about your cancer
- stay away from you, or keep their visits short

Finding a Good Listener

It can be hard to talk about how it feels to have cancer. But talking can help, even though it is hard to do. Many people find that they feel better when they share their thoughts and feelings with their close family and friends.

Friends and family members may not always know what to say to you. Sometimes they can help by just being good listeners. They don't always need to give you advice or tell you what they think. They simply need to show that they care and are concerned about you.

You might find it helpful to talk about your feelings with people who are not family or friends. Instead, you might want to meet in a support group with others who have cancer or talk with a counselor. You can find more information about where to go for help in Chapter 5, "People Helping People" starting on page 37.

> A single arrow is easily broken, but not ten in a bundle.
> —*Japanese Proverb*

Choosing a Good Time to Talk

Some people need time before they can talk about their feelings. If you are not ready, you might say, "I don't feel like talking about my cancer right now." And sometimes when you want to talk, your family and friends may not be ready to listen.

It is hard for other people to know when to talk about cancer. Sometimes people send a signal when they want to talk. They might:

- bring up the subject of cancer
- talk about things that have to do with cancer, such as a newspaper story about a new cancer treatment that they just read
- spend more time with you
- act nervous or make jokes that aren't very funny

You can help people feel more comfortable by asking them what they think or how they feel. Sometimes people can't put their feelings into words. Sometimes, they just want to hug each other or cry together. A man with stomach cancer said,

"It was really hard to get my sister to talk about my cancer. Finally, I just said to her, 'I know you're really worried and scared. So am I. Let's talk about it.' She was so relieved that I had brought the subject up."

Expressing Anger

Many people feel angry or frustrated when they deal with cancer. You might find that you get mad or upset with the people you depend on. You may get upset with small things that never bothered you before.

People can't always express their feelings. Anger sometimes shows up as actions instead of words. You may find that you yell a lot at the kids or the dog. You might slam doors.

Try to figure out why you are angry. Maybe you are afraid of the cancer or are worried about money. You might even be angry about your treatment. A man with advanced cancer said,

"I got so angry some days that I just wanted to take it out on something. On those days, I always tried to be angry at my cancer, not at my wife and daughter."

When anger rises, think of the consequences.
—*Confucius*

Pretending to Be Cheerful

Some people pretend to be cheerful, even when they are not. They think that they will not feel sad or angry when they act cheerful. Your family and friends may not want to upset you and will act as if nothing is bothering them. You may think that by being cheerful, your cancer will go away.

When you have cancer, you have many reasons to be upset. "Down days" are to be expected. Don't pretend to be cheerful when you're not. This can keep you from getting the help you need. Be honest and talk about all your feelings, not just the cheerful ones. An older woman with liver cancer said,

"The advice of well-meaning friends to be positive, optimistic, and upbeat can also be a call for silence. Ask them about it. Don't let them force you to put on a fake smile when that's the last thing you feel like doing."

Sharing Without Talking

For many, it's hard to talk about being sick. Others feel that cancer is a personal or private matter and find it hard to talk openly about it. If talking is hard for you, think about other ways to share your feelings. For instance, you may find it helpful to write about your feelings. This might be a good time to start a journal or diary if you don't already have one. Writing about your feelings is a good way to sort through them and a good way to begin to deal with them. All you need to get started is something to write with and something to write on.

Journals can be personal or shared. People can use a journal as a way of 'talking' to each other. If you find it hard to talk to someone near to you about your cancer try starting a shared journal. Leave a booklet or pad in a private place that both of you select. When you need to share, write in it and return it to the private place. Your loved one will do the same. Both of you will be able to know how the other is feeling without having to speak aloud.

If you have e-mail, this can also be a good way to share without talking.

Summing Up: Sharing Your Thoughts and Feelings About Cancer

Cancer is hard to deal with all alone. Although talking about your cancer can be hard at first, most people find that sharing their thoughts and feelings helps them deal with their cancer.

Keep in mind:

- **Choose a good listener.** You may not need someone to give you advice or tell you what to do. Instead, you may want someone who wants to hear about and try to understand what life is like for you right now. You may need to look outside your family to find such a person.

- **Choose a good time to share.** Sometimes people will send signals to let you know they are willing to talk about cancer with you. Sometimes you can ask others about their thoughts and feelings.

- **Understand anger.** Sometimes angry words come from emotions other than anger, like frustration, worry, or sadness. Try to figure out why you feel angry and why you need to express it. Don't run away from these feelings—share them and try to understand them.

- **Don't pretend to be cheerful.** You may want to spare those around you from your strong feelings, but acting cheerful will not help you express your true feelings. Acting cheerful will not give others a true picture of your thoughts and feelings.

- **Turn to community resources for help.** A support group or a counselor might be able to provide more support.

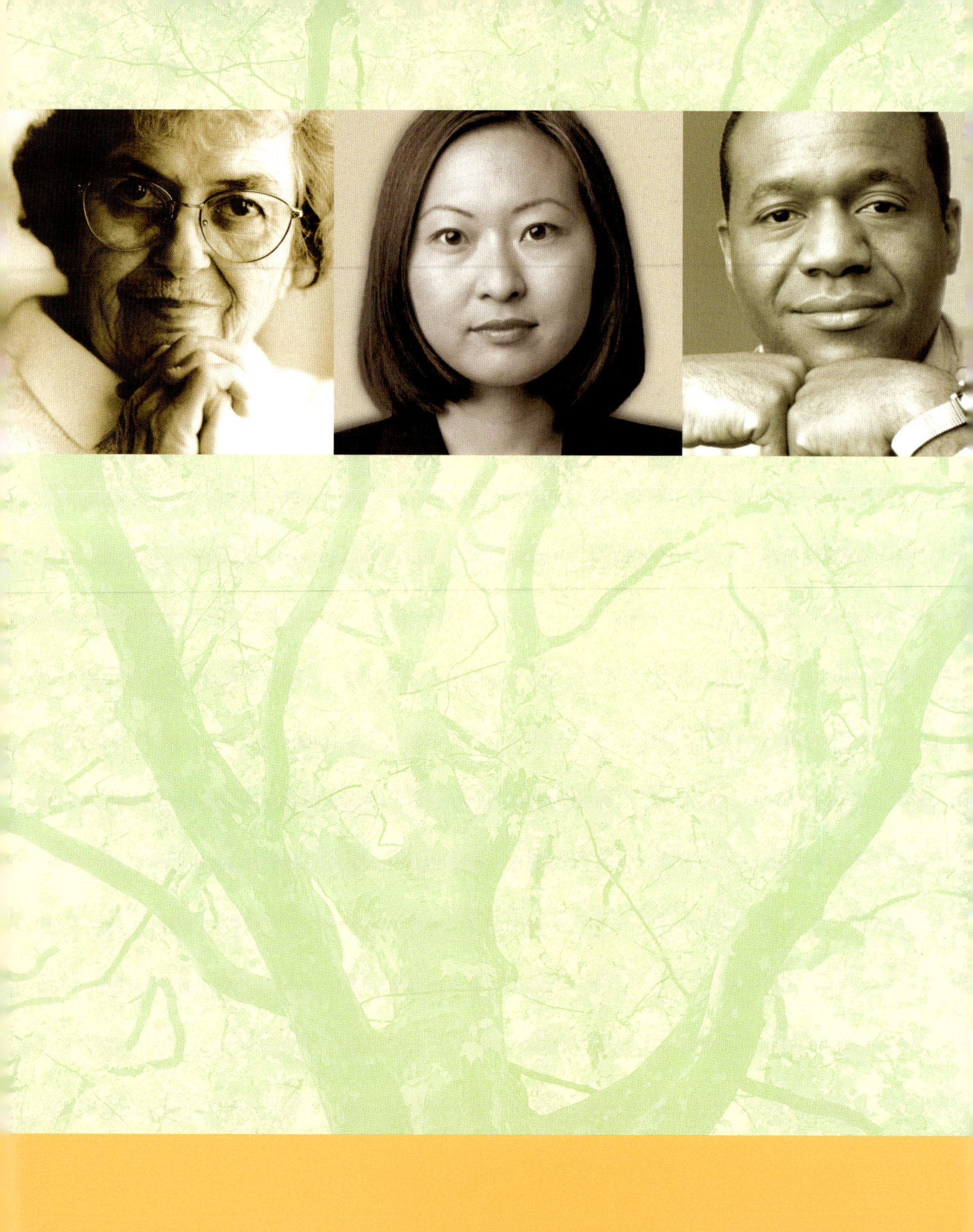

CHAPTER 4

Learning About Your Cancer and Feeling More in Control

When you first learn you have cancer, daily life can feel like it is turned upside down. Learning more about your type of cancer and its treatment can help you feel more in control.

Learn about your type of cancer and its treatment by:

- asking your doctor or nurse questions
- taking notes during your doctor visits
- getting a second opinion
- calling the Cancer Information Service at 1-800-422-6237
- looking up your type of cancer on the Internet at http://cancer.gov
- visiting a public library or a hospital library for patients and families

Learning about your cancer can help you talk to your doctor about which treatment is right for you.

"At first, I felt overwhelmed. But once I gathered information, I felt comfortable talking with my doctor about my cancer and ready to make decisions about my treatment."

Cancer can rob people of a sense of control over their lives. You may feel that your future is uncertain and you do not know if you will live or die. Or you may rely on doctors you hardly know to help you make health decisions.

People often feel more in control when they learn as much as they can about cancer and its treatment. They say that it is easier to make decisions when they know what to expect. How much do you know about your cancer and its treatment?

> **When you see clouds gathering, prepare to catch rainwater.**
> —*Gola (African) Proverb*

Learning From Your Health Care Providers

Doctors, nurses, and other health care providers can teach you a lot about cancer and its treatment. But sometimes people have trouble learning because they are scared or confused. These feelings can make it hard to learn new information. But, there are things you can do to make it easier to learn.

Ask your doctor or nurse to write down the name and stage of your cancer.

There are many different types of cancer and each type has its own name. "Stage" refers to the size of the cancer tumor and how far it has spread in your body. Knowing the name and stage of your cancer will help:

- you find out more about your cancer
- your doctor and you decide what treatment choices you have

Ask as many questions as you need to.

Your doctor needs to know your questions and concerns. Write down your questions and bring them with you to the doctor's visit. Sometimes you can even send your questions ahead of time. Your doctor can get information ready for you if he or she knows your questions in advance. If you have a lot of questions, you and your doctor may want to plan extra time to talk about them.

Don't worry if your questions seem silly or don't make sense.

All your questions are important and deserve an answer. It's okay to ask the same question more than once. It's also okay to ask your doctor to use simpler words and explain terms that are new to you. To make sure you understand, use your own words to repeat back what you heard the doctor say.

> **One who asks is a fool for five minutes, but one who does not ask remains a fool forever.**
> —*Chinese Proverb*

Take someone along when you see the doctor.

Ask a family member or friend to go with you when you see your doctor. This person can help by listening, taking notes, and asking questions. Later, you can both talk about what the doctor had to say. If you can't find someone to go with you when you see the doctor, ask your doctor if he or she will talk with a friend or family member over the phone.

Take notes or tape record your conversation with your doctor.

Many patients have trouble remembering what they talk about with their doctor. Ask if you can take notes or make a tape recording. Review these notes or listen to the tape later. This can help you remember what you talked about. You might also want to let your family and friends see these notes so that they, too, can learn what the doctor had to say.

Learning About Your Treatment Choices

You can learn about your treatment choices by:

- asking your doctor
- getting a second opinion
- calling the Cancer Information Service (see page 34)
- reading about your type of cancer on the Internet

> Every road has two directions.
> —*Russian Proverb*

Ask Your Doctor to tell you about your treatment choices. Sometimes there is more than one treatment that can help. Ask how each treatment can help and what side effects (reactions to the treatment) you might have. If your doctor asks you to choose which treatment you want, try to learn all you can about each choice. Let your doctor know if you need more time to think about these issues before your treatment begins.

Get a Second Opinion from a doctor who takes care of cancer patients (an oncologist). The oncologist may agree with your first doctor's treatment plan. Or he or she may suggest something else. Many health insurance plans pay for a second opinion. Read your policy, call your insurance company, or speak with a social worker to learn if your insurance plan will pay for a second opinion.

Call the Cancer Information Service at 1-800-4-CANCER (1-800-422-6237) or TTY (for deaf and hard of hearing callers) at 1-800-332-8615. They can answer questions and send you information about treatment choices for different kinds of cancer.

Read About Your Type of Cancer on the National Cancer Institute Web site at **http://cancer.gov**

Learning More About Your Cancer

There are many other ways to learn about your cancer. You can read books or journal articles or search for information on the Internet. Make sure, however, to talk with your doctor about what you learn. He or she can explain what you don't understand and let you know if anything is untrue or not useful for you. Here are some ways to get more information about cancer:

- Ask your doctor for printed materials (such as booklets or fact sheets) about your type of cancer or about cancer in general.

- Look for cancer information at your public library or visit a library for patients and family members at your local hospital or medical school.

- Call your hospital and ask if they have cancer programs for patients and family members. Many hospitals offer classes and support groups.

- Search the Internet. The National Cancer Institute Web site at **http://cancer.gov** is a good place to start. If you do not have a computer at home, most public libraries have computers you can use.

- Contact the Cancer Information Service (see above).

Summing Up: Learning About Your Cancer and Regaining Control

When you find out you have cancer, you may feel that your life is no longer within your control. As if daily life is turned upside down.

For many people, regaining a sense of control begins by learning as much as they can about their cancer. Talk to your doctor and nurses. Seek information from the library, the Internet, and the Cancer Information Service to help you learn about your type of cancer and its treatment.

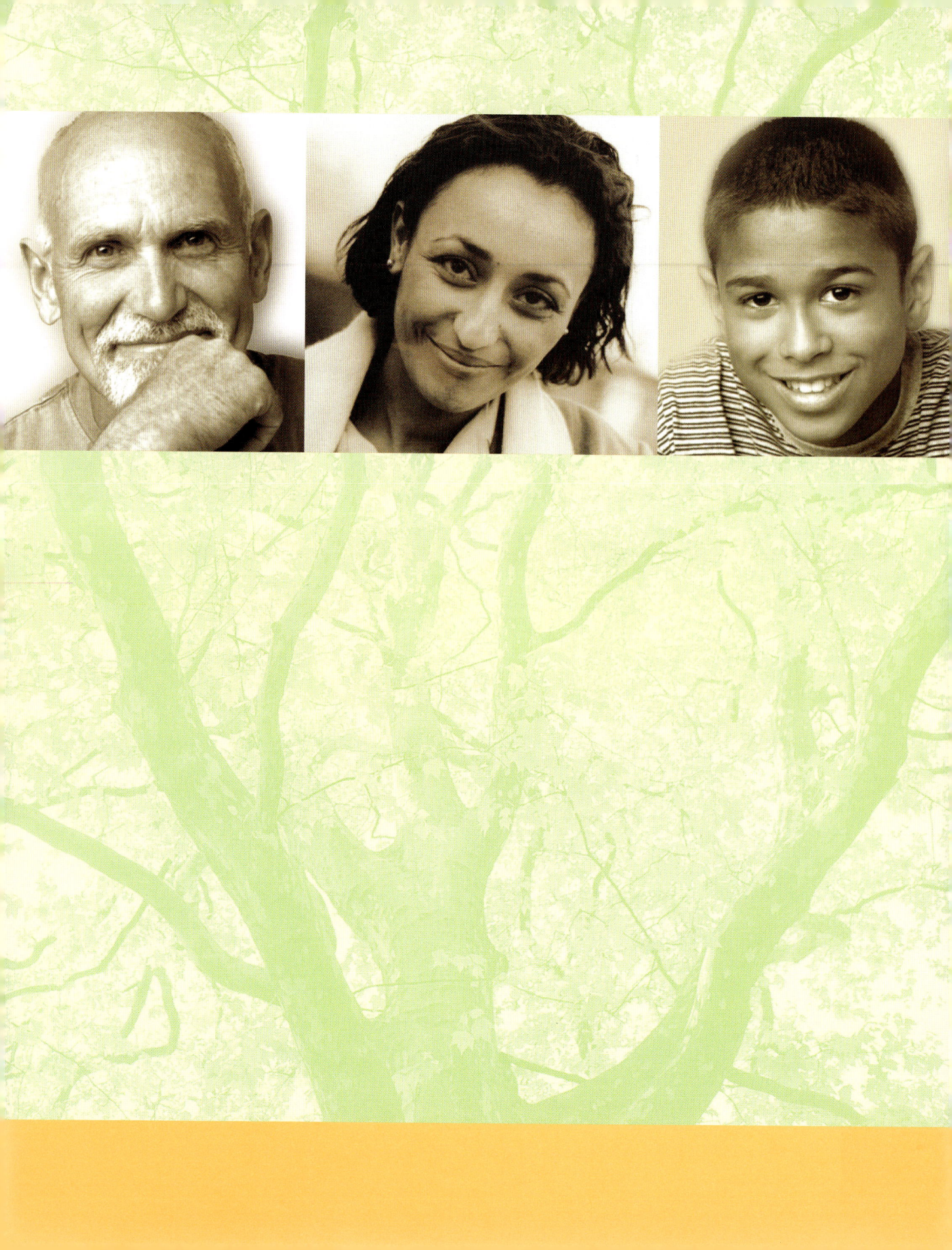

CHAPTER 5

People Helping People

Even though your needs are greater when you have cancer, it can be hard to ask for help to meet those needs.

To get the help you need, think about turning to:

- family and friends
- others who also have cancer
- people you meet in support groups
- people from your spiritual or religious community
- health care providers
- caregivers

No one needs to face cancer alone. When people with cancer seek and receive help from others, they often find it easier to cope.

You may find it hard to ask for or accept help. After all, you are used to taking care of yourself. Maybe you think that asking for help is a sign of weakness. Or perhaps you do not want to let others know that some things are hard for you to do. All these feelings are normal. As one man with cancer said:

"I had always been the strong one. Now I had to turn to others for help. It wasn't easy at first, but the support of others helped me get through a lot of hard times."

People feel good when they help others. Your friends may not know what to say or how to act when they are with you. Some people may even avoid you. But they may feel more at ease when you ask them to cook a meal or pick up your children after school. There are many ways that family, friends, other people who have cancer, spiritual or religious leaders, and health care providers can help. In turn, there are also ways you can help and support your caregivers.

Family and Friends

Family and friends can support you in many ways. But, they may wait for you to give them hints or ideas about what to do. Someone who is not sure if you want company may call "just to see how things are going." When someone says, "Let me know if there is anything I can do," tell this person if you need help with an errand or a ride to the doctor's office.

Family members and friends can also:

- keep you company, give you a hug, or hold your hand
- listen as you talk about your hopes and fears
- help with rides, meals, errands, or household chores
- go with you to doctor's visits or treatment sessions
- tell other friends and family members ways they can help

> A little help is better than a lot of pity.
> —*Celtic Proverb*

Other People Who Have Cancer

Even though your family and friends help, you may also want to meet people who have cancer now or have had it in the past. Often, you can talk with them about things you can't discuss with others. People with cancer understand how you feel and can:

- talk with you about what to expect
- tell you how they cope with cancer and live a normal life
- help you learn ways to enjoy each day
- give you hope for the future

Let your doctor or nurse know that you want to meet other people with cancer. You can also meet other people with cancer in the hospital, at your doctor's office, or through a cancer support group.

> To know the road ahead, ask those coming back.
> —Chinese Proverb

Support Groups

Cancer support groups are meetings for people with cancer and those touched by cancer. These groups allow you and your loved ones to talk with others facing the same problems. Support groups often have a lecture as well as time to talk. Almost all groups have a leader who runs the meeting. The leader can be someone with cancer or a trained counselor.

You may think that a support group is not right for you. Maybe you think that a group won't help or that you don't want to talk with others about your feelings. Or perhaps you are afraid that the meetings will make you sad or depressed.

It may be good to know that many people find support groups very helpful. People in the groups often:

- talk about what it's like to have cancer
- help each other feel better, more hopeful, and not so alone
- learn about what's new in cancer treatment
- share tips about ways to cope with cancer

As one woman said,

"I can't tell you what a pleasure it was when I first sat down with other cancer patients and heard my own fears, furies, and joys coming from their lips. You can be completely honest with these people. I'd leave some of these sessions almost dizzy with relief."

Types of Support Groups

- Some groups focus on all kinds of cancer. Others talk about just one kind, such as a group for women with breast cancer or a group for men with prostate cancer.

- Groups can be open to everyone or just for people of a certain age, sex, culture, or religion. For instance, some groups are just for teens or young children.

- Some groups talk about all aspects of cancer. Others focus on only one or two topics such as treatment choices or self-esteem.

- Therapy groups focus on feelings such as sadness and grief. Mental Health professionals often lead these types of groups. (See "People in Health Care" starting on page 42.)

- In some groups, people with cancer meet in one support group and their loved ones meet in another. This way, people can say what they really think and feel and not worry about hurting someone's feelings.

- In other groups, patients and families meet together. People often find that meeting in these groups is a good way for each to learn what the other is going through.

- Online support groups are "meetings" that take place by computer. People meet through chat rooms, listservs, or moderated discussion groups and talk with each other over e-mail. People often like online support groups because they can take part in them any time of the day or night. They're also good for people who can't travel to meetings. The biggest problem with online groups is that you can't be sure if what you learn is correct. Always talk with your doctor about cancer information you learn from the Internet.

If you have a choice of support groups, visit a few and see what they are like. See which ones make sense for you. Although many groups are free, some charge a small fee. Find out if your health insurance pays for support groups.

Where to Find a Support Group

Many hospitals, cancer centers, community groups, and schools offer cancer support groups. Here are some ways to find groups near you:

- Call your local hospital and ask about its cancer support programs.

- Look in the health section of your local newspaper for a listing of cancer support groups.

Spiritual Help

Spirituality means the way you look at the world and make sense of your place in it. Spirituality can include faith or religion, beliefs, values, and "reasons for being."

Most people are spiritual in some way, whether or not they go to a church, temple, or mosque.

Cancer can affect people's spirituality. Some people find that cancer brings a new or deeper meaning to their faith. Others feel that their faith has let them down. For example, you may:

- struggle to understand why you have cancer
- wonder about life's purpose and how cancer fits in the "fabric of life"
- question your relationship with God

Many people find that their faith is a source of comfort. They find they can cope better with cancer when they pray, read religious books, meditate, or talk with members of their spiritual community. The wife of a man with cancer said,

"I could not handle my husband's illness on my own. It's real hard when I have my down times. But my faith gives me strength and, mostly, I have peace about it."

Many people also find that cancer changes their values. The things you own and your daily duties may seem less important. You may decide to spend more time with loved ones, helping others, doing things in the outdoors, or learning about something new.

One who is contented is not always rich.
—Spanish Proverb

People in Health Care

Most cancer patients have a treatment team of health providers who work together to help them. This team may include doctors, nurses, social workers, pharmacists, dietitians, and other people in health care. Chances are that you will never see all these people at the same time. In fact, there may be health providers on your team who you never meet.

Doctors

Most people with cancer have two or more doctors. Chances are, you will see one doctor most often. This person is the leader of your team. He or she not only meets with you but also works with all the other people on your treatment team.

Make sure to let your doctor know how you are feeling. Tell him or her when you feel sick, are depressed, or in pain. (To learn more, read about "Pain Scales and Pain Journals" on page 5). When your doctor knows how you feel, he or she can:

- figure out if you are getting better or worse
- decide if you need other drugs or treatments
- help you get the extra support you need

Ask your doctor how often he or she will see you, when you will have tests, and how long before you know if the treatment is working.

Nurses

Most likely, you will see nurses more often than other people on your treatment team. If you are in the hospital, nurses will check in on you many times a day. If you are at home, visiting nurses may come to your house and help with your treatment and care. Nurses also work in clinics and doctor offices.

You can talk with nurses about your day-to-day concerns. They can tell you what to expect, such as if a certain drug is likely to make you feel sick. You can also talk with nurses about what worries you. They can offer hope, support, and suggest ways to talk with family and friends about your feelings.

Nurses work with all the other health providers on your treatment team. Let them know if you need or want more help.

Pharmacists

Pharmacists not only fill prescriptions but also can teach you about the drugs you are taking. They can help you by:

- talking with you about how your drugs work
- telling you how often to take your drugs
- teaching you about side effects and how to deal with them
- warning you about the danger of mixing drugs together
- letting you know about foods you shouldn't eat or things you shouldn't do, like being in the sun for too long

Dietitians

People with cancer often have trouble eating or digesting food. Eating problems can be a side effect from cancer drugs or treatments. They can also happen when people are so upset that they lose their appetite and don't feel like eating.

Dietitians can help by teaching you about foods that are healthy, taste good, and are easy to eat. They can also suggest ways to make eating easier, such as using plastic forks or spoons so food doesn't taste like metal when you are having chemo. Ask your doctor or nurse to refer you to a dietitian who knows about the special needs of cancer patients.

Social Workers

Social workers assist patients and families with meeting their daily needs such as:

- finding support groups near where you live
- dealing with money matters, like paying the bills
- talking about your cancer with your boss
- filling out paperwork, such as advance directives or living wills (For more information about advance directives and living wills, see Chapter 7 "Living Each Day" on page 63.)
- talking about your cancer with your family and other loved ones
- dealing with your feelings such as depression, sadness, or grief

- coping with stress and learning new ways to relax
- learning about health insurance, such as what your policy covers and what it does not
- finding rides to the hospital, clinic, or doctor's office
- setting up visits from home health nurses

Patient Educators

Patient or health educators can help you learn more about your cancer. They can find information that fits your needs. Patient educators are also experts in explaining things that may be hard to understand. Many hospitals and treatment centers have resource centers run by health educators. These centers contain books, videos, computers, and other tools to help you and your family. These tools can help you understand your type of cancer, your treatment choices, side effects, and tips for living with and beyond your cancer. Ask your doctor or nurse about talking to a patient educator.

Psychologists

Most people are very upset when they face a serious illness such as cancer. Psychologists can help by talking with you and your family about your worries. They can not only help you figure out what upsets you but also teach you ways to cope with these feelings and concerns.

Let your doctor or nurse know if you want to talk with a psychologist who is trained to help people with cancer.

Psychiatrists

Sometimes people with cancer are depressed or have other psychiatric (mental health) disorders. Psychiatrists are medical doctors who can prescribe drugs for these disorders. They can also talk with you about your feelings and help you find the mental health services you need.

Let your doctor know if you feel like you need to meet with a psychiatrist.

Licensed Counselors and Other Mental Health Professionals

Licensed counselors, pastoral care professionals, spiritual leaders, nurse practitioners, and other mental health professionals also help people deal with their feelings, worries, and concerns. For instance, they can:

- help you talk about feelings such as stress, depression, or grief
- lead support groups and therapy sessions
- act as a "go-between," such as with your child's school or your boss at work
- refer you to other health providers and services near where you live

Talk with your doctor or contact your local cancer center to find mental health professionals near you.

People in the Hospital

Many hospitals have people on staff to help make your stay a little easier.

Patient advocates can help when you have a problem or concern that you don't feel you can discuss with your doctor, nurse, or social worker. They can act as a bridge between you and your health care team.

Discharge planners work with you and your family to help you get ready to leave the hospital. The discharge planner helps with tasks like making follow-up appointments and making sure you have things you need at home.

Volunteers often visit with patients in the hospital and offer comfort and support. They may also bring books, puzzles, or other things to do. Many volunteers have had cancer themselves. Let a hospital staff member know if you want to meet with a volunteer.

Caregivers

Caregivers are the people who help with your daily tasks such as bathing, getting dressed, or eating. Caregivers are often family members or close friends. Just like you, your caregivers need help and support. Ways to help your caregiver include:

- building a team
- keeping your caregivers informed
- finding extra help
- doing what you can to help your caregiver
- showing your caregiver that you care

> There is no one-way friendship.
> —Maasai (African) Proverb

Build a Team

Build a team of caregivers so that you don't have to depend on just one person. With a team, people can take turns with tasks such as:

- washing your hair or giving you a backrub
- going food shopping or cooking a meal for you
- driving you to the doctor's office
- doing errands like going to the bank or post office
- cleaning the kitchen or mowing your lawn
- picking up your children after school

Keep Your Caregivers Informed

Make sure your caregivers know about your treatment and care. Ask your doctor or nurse to talk with the person who helps you the most. Suggest they talk about your cancer and its treatment and also what to do in case of an emergency.

You can help by:

- **Making a list of important phone numbers.** This list should have the phone numbers of your doctor, nurse, pharmacist, family members, neighbors, friends, and spiritual leaders. Keep copies of this list next to each phone in your house.

- **Letting your caregivers know about the drugs you take.** Make an up-to-date list of all your drugs. Include the name of each drug, as well as how much of this drug you take and how often you need to take it. Be sure to also let your caregivers know about side effects to watch for and if you have any drug allergies.

- **Telling your caregivers about important paperwork.** Let your caregivers know where you keep a copy of your insurance policies, social security papers, living will or advance directive, and power of attorney form. (For more information about advance directives, living wills, and power of attorney see Chapter 7 "Living Each Day" on page 63.)

Find Help Where You Live

Many towns have community volunteers. These people offer help to others near where they live or work. Here are some ways to find volunteers:

- Look in your local newspaper.
- Ask at your hospital, library, or place of worship.
- Call your state or local health department.
- Contact the Cancer Information Service (see "Resources for Learning More" on page 65.) and ask how to find volunteer programs near you.

Some towns also have services such as respite care, home care, and hospice.

Respite Care programs arrange for someone else to stay with you while your caregivers take time off. To learn more about respite care, call your local hospital, home care agency, or hospice program. For ways to find out more, see "Resources for Learning More" on page 65.

Home Care programs arrange for you to receive skilled nursing care or help with personal tasks such as bathing or dressing in your own home. Your doctor needs to order these services. Talk with your doctor or nurse if you want to learn more.

Hospice can be a great source of comfort and support to people who are dying. It can help with medical care and be a way for people who are dying and their families to talk about their feelings. In some towns, hospice can also help with respite care. Let your doctor know if you want to learn more about a hospice near you.

> When you have no choice, mobilize the spirit of courage.
> —*Jewish Proverb*

Take Care of Your Caregivers

Cancer and its treatment are hard on everyone, even the people who take care of you. Encourage your caregivers to take time off so they can do errands, enjoy hobbies, or simply have a rest.

Your caregivers might want to join a support group and meet others who are also caring for people with cancer. To find a group nearby, contact your local hospital or cancer center.

Watch for signs of depression in your caregivers. If you think that one of them is depressed, talk to him or her about it. Urge your caregiver to seek professional help. Let him or her know that other people can help you while they are taking care of themselves. To learn more about the signs of depression, see page 8.

Show That You Care

Try to keep your sense of humor. If you like to joke with your friends and family, don't stop now. It's okay to laugh at things that make you upset. For many people, humor is a way to gain a sense of control. A woman who just had cancer surgery said,

"I had a lot of tubes and such hooked up to me after my surgery, and I could tell it made some of my visitors uncomfortable. When I noticed them staring at all the high-tech stuff, I'd make a joke about being the 'Bionic Woman.' They'd laugh at that and relax, and then we'd be able to talk."

> One kind word can warm three winter months.
> —*Japanese Proverb*

And remember to say "thank you." Let your caregivers know that you value their help, support, and love.

Summing Up: People Helping People

People who have cancer often find that their needs change because of their cancer. The tasks of daily life become harder to manage. Feelings can be intense. And spiritual questions loom larger than ever before.

Even though their needs are greater, it is hard for many people with cancer to ask for help. Many people do not know where to look for the help they need.

People you can turn to for help include:

- **Family and friends.** Most people are happy to find out that something they have to offer—a meal, a ride to the doctor, a phone call—is helpful to you. They may want to offer you help but do not know what you need or want.

- **Others who also have cancer.** People who have been through cancer often share a special bond with one another. Sharing what you have been through with others and hearing how they have coped can be a source of strength for you.

- **Support groups.** There are many types of groups. Think about what you would like in a group and talk to your health care provider to help you find that type of group.

- **Spiritual help,** which can come from your church, synagogue, or other religious center. Or you may find that reading, talking with others, and meditating or praying provide you with a sense of peace and strength.

- **Health care providers** both in the community and in the hospital. A whole range of specially trained people are available to help you meet all your needs.

- **Caregivers,** who provide your day-to-day care. As they care for you, remind them that they need to care for their own needs as well.

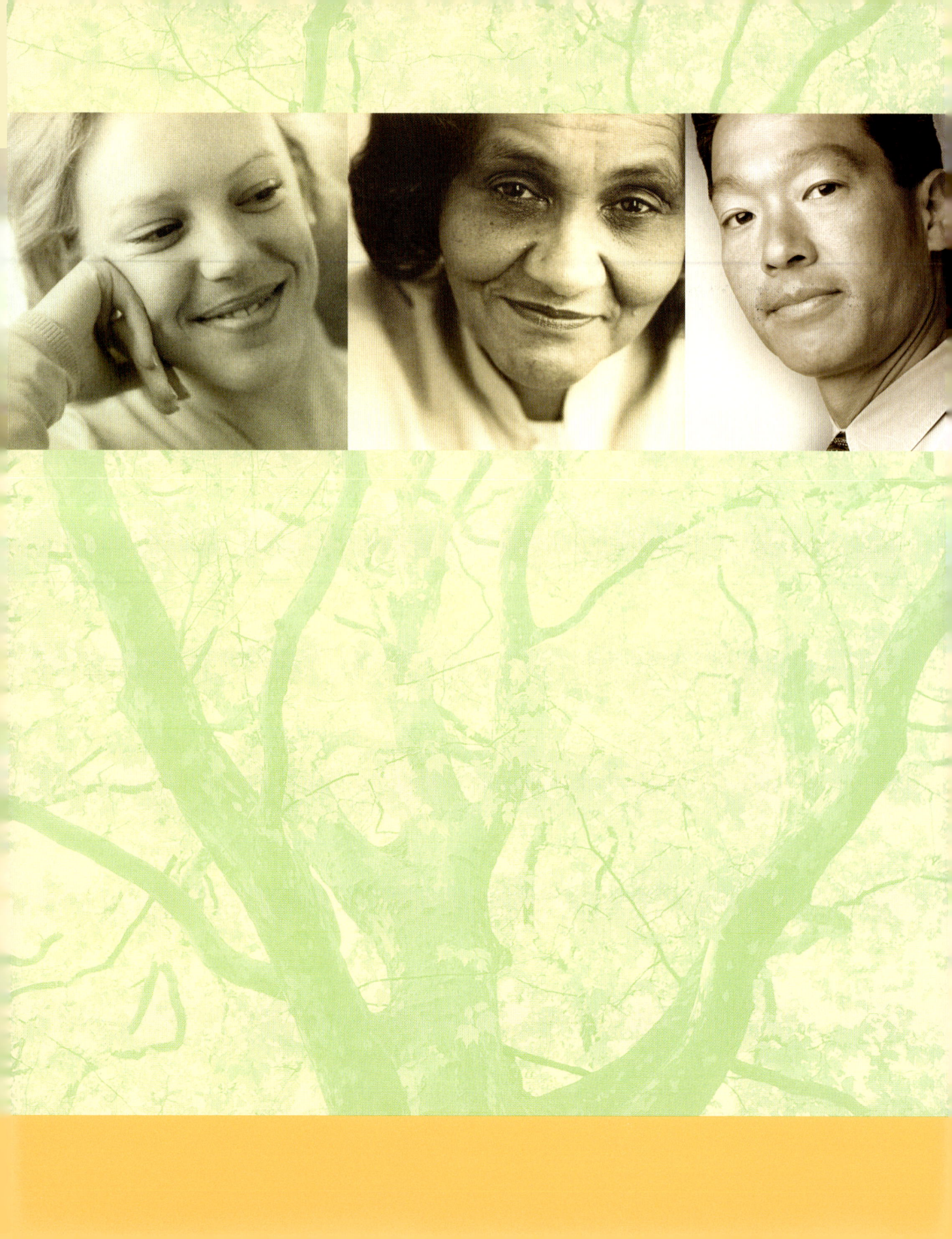

CHAPTER 6

Dealing With a New Self-Image

When you have cancer and when you are having treatment for cancer, changes occur.

- You don't have as much energy as you did before the cancer.
- Your body is not the same as it was.
- If you're single, your dating life may be awkward. You may face new challenges in your sex life.
- If you have a partner, you may face changes in your relationship.

These changes can be hard to accept. But most people with cancer find that, with time, they are able to develop a new self-image by:

- staying actively involved in life
- getting help when they need it
- talking openly about sex and intimacy with their loved ones

Cancer and its treatment can change how you look and feel.

- Surgery can leave scars or change the way you look.
- Chemotherapy can cause your hair to fall out.
- Radiation can make you feel very tired.
- Some drugs may cause you to gain weight or feel bloated.
- Treatments can make it hard to eat. They may upset your stomach and make you throw up. Or they can make you feel so sick that you do not want to eat.
- Some treatments can make it hard to get pregnant or father a child.

Cancer treatment can last for weeks or months. The good news is that most of these side effects go away when the treatment is over.

Many people want to know as much as they can about side effects, even before treatment begins. This way, they can talk with their doctor about ways to treat them. For example, a doctor can change a person's drugs or suggest new foods to eat.

If you think you might want to have children in the future, ask your doctor to refer you to a fertility doctor before you begin treatment for your cancer.

Fatigue

Many people feel fatigue (they are very tired or have little energy) when they are being treated for cancer. They may have good days with lots of energy and bad days when they are very tired. This fatigue is likely to last for a while after treatment is over. For some people, it can last for many months.

Let people know that you have both good and bad days. Try to do something special on days when you feel better. Let yourself rest on the days you are very tired. And don't be afraid to tell others if you feel fatigue, even if you need to change your plans.

"Before my cancer, I was always full of energy, working full-time, coming home to family activities, playing tennis, and enjoying an active social life. Now, I have to conserve my energy and plan my schedule around my chemotherapy. Many days I am so tired, it's an effort to just get out of bed."

Your Self-Image

Each of us has a mental picture of how we look, our "self-image." Although we may not always like how we look, we are used to and accept our self-image.

Cancer and its treatment can change your self-image. You may have changes such as hair loss or scars from surgery. Some of these changes (hair loss) will go away when treatment is over. Other changes (scars) will always be a part of how you look. Every person changes in different ways. Some changes people will notice and other changes only you will notice. Some changes you may like and with some others, you may need time to adjust.

Coping with these changes can be hard. But, over time, most people learn to accept them. Your family and friends can help by showing they love you the way you are.

Staying Active

Many people find that staying active can help. Whether you swim, play a sport, or take an exercise class, you may find that being active helps you accept your new self-image. Talk with your doctor about ways you can stay active.

Hobbies and volunteer work can also help improve your self-image. You may like to read, listen to music, or sew. You may also want to teach a child how to read or volunteer at a homeless shelter. You may find that you feel better about yourself when you get involved in helping others and doing things you enjoy.

Getting Help

Reconstructive surgery. If cancer surgery changes the way you look, you may want to have reconstructive surgery (plastic surgery). Many patients feel that this type of surgery helps them cope better with their new self-image. For instance, you may choose to have surgery to improve the look of a surgical scar. Most insurance companies pay for reconstructive surgery.

Prosthetic devices. If a part of your body needs to be amputated (cut off) because of cancer, a prosthetic device (a fake or man-made body part) can replace what was cut off. For example, if your leg is amputated, you may want to have a prosthetic leg to replace the one you lost. Most insurance companies pay for prosthetic devices.

Wigs and scarves. Cancer treatment may cause you to lose your hair. You may want to cover your head to keep you warm and protected from the sun. You may also feel that wearing a wig or scarf improves how you look.

It is a good idea to buy your wig before treatment starts. This way, the wig will match the color and style of your own hair. You may want to start wearing your wig before losing your hair. Try to find a wig or scarf that fits well and is not scratchy, since your scalp may be tender and sore. You may be able to deduct the cost of your wig from your income taxes. Most of the time, your hair will grow back when treatment is over, even though it may be a different color and not feel like it did before.

Facing Cancer With Your Spouse or Partner

Some couples grow stronger when they face cancer together. They look at their lives in a new way. Problems that once seemed big don't feel that way now. Other couples facing cancer have more trouble. A psychologist said,

"If a couple had a good relationship before cancer treatment, they have a good basis for dealing with new problems. If the relationship has problems, the real reasons for these problems were probably there before the cancer."

Your Sex Life May Change

Sometimes people with cancer and their partners or spouses have trouble showing their love for each other. For instance, one man said that his wife wouldn't kiss him any more because she was afraid that she would catch cancer. In truth, people cannot give each other cancer. If your loved one is worried about catching cancer from you, suggest he or she talk with your doctor.

People can also have problems with sex because of cancer and its treatment. For instance, you may not like how you look and not want to have sex. If this happens, talk with your spouse or partner. Your partner probably loves you for more than your body. A 45-year-old man said,

"My wife found it hard to understand that my love for her wasn't less because she had a mastectomy. I was much more concerned that she be rid of the cancer. I had to convince her that I loved her for her many special qualities, not her left breast."

Your spouse or partner may be afraid to have sex with you. He or she may be afraid of hurting you or having sex when you are not feeling well. Let your partner know if you want to have sex or would rather just hug, kiss, and cuddle.

Sometimes, cancer and its treatment causes other problems with sex.

- Fatigue can make you so tired that you don't want to have sex.
- Surgery can make certain positions painful.
- Prostate cancer treatments can make it hard for a man to have an erection.
- Some treatments cause women to have vaginal dryness.
- Orgasm is sometimes hard to achieve.

Even though you may feel awkward, talk about your sex life with people who can help. Let your doctor or nurse know if you are having problems. There may be drugs you can take or other ways you and your loved one can give each other pleasure. Some people also find it helpful to talk with other couples about how to stay close while dealing with cancer.

Remember that you are special for who you are, not how you look. Your sense of humor, intellect, sweetness, common sense, special talents, and loyalty, these and many other qualities make you special. Sex is not the only basis for a relationship. It is one of many ways to express love and respect.

Dating

If you are single, you may worry about dating. You may be afraid that you are not as good looking as you used to be. And you may not know how, or when, to talk with someone new about your cancer.

One woman with breast cancer said that dating was easier than she thought it would be. She felt like she knew when the time was right to talk about her disease. In fact, she said that her cancer never caused problems with people she dated.

"I told my boyfriend about my breast cancer and my reluctance to let him see my body. He was very reassuring. He said it didn't matter to him— that I was important for who I was, not how my body looked."

Summing Up: Dealing With a New Self-Image

When you have cancer and when you are having treatment for cancer, you go through changes.

- You don't have as much energy as you did before the cancer.

- Your body is not the same as it was.

- If you're single, your dating life may be awkward.

- You may face new problems in your sex life.

These changes can be hard to accept. But most people with cancer find that, with time, they learn to accept their new self-image by:

- staying involved in life

- getting help when they need it

- talking openly about sex and feelings of closeness with their loved ones

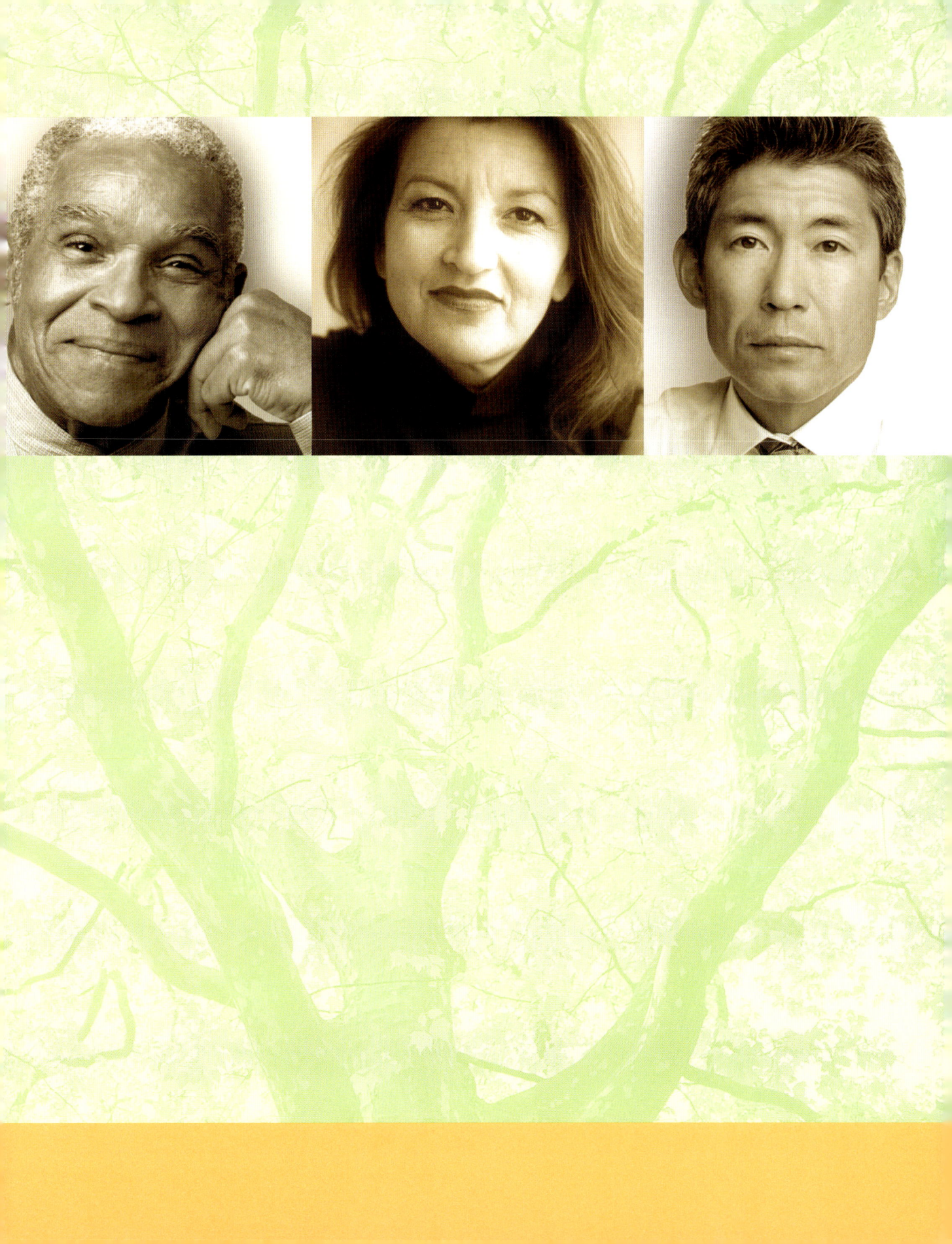

CHAPTER 7

Living Each Day

When you have cancer, living each day to the fullest means:

- staying involved in the duties and pleasures of daily life
- returning to work if possible
- making plans for the future

Is living with cancer the biggest challenge you have ever faced? For most people, it is. Dealing with cancer and facing thoughts of death is a life-changing event for most people.

"My cancer made me take a closer look at how I spend my days. Realizing that they might be limited, I was determined to make them as good as possible. I vowed to use my time in ways that were good for me or brought me pleasure."

Try to live each day as normally as you can. Enjoy the simple things you like to do such as petting your cat or watching a sunset. Take pleasure in big events such as a friend's wedding or your grandson's high school graduation.

> Every season brings its own joy.
> —*Spanish proverb*

Keeping Up With Your Daily Routine

If you feel well enough, keep up with your daily routine. This includes going to work, spending time with family and friends, taking part in hobbies, and even going on trips.

At the same time, give yourself time to be with your feelings about cancer. Also, be careful about acting cheerful when you are not. Avoiding your feelings may make you feel worse, not better. (To learn more, go to Chapter 3 on page 25, "Sharing Your Feelings About Cancer.")

Use these questions to think about how you want to spend your time.

- Who do I like to be with?
- Who makes me laugh?
- How do I want to spend my time?
- What makes me feel happy?
- What types of things do I enjoy the most?
- What types of things do I like the least?
- Is there something I want to do that I've never tried?

Fun

Sometimes people with cancer try new, fun things that they have never done before. For instance, have you always wanted to ride in a hot air balloon or go deep-sea fishing? What fun things have you always wanted to try, but have never taken the time to do? A young woman with cancer put it this way,

"Too often we patients fill up our lives with meaningful activities and neglect the frivolous outlets that keep us sane."

Try to do something just for fun, not because you have to do it. But be careful not to tire yourself out. Some people get depressed when they are too tired. Make sure to get enough rest so you feel strong and can enjoy these fun activities.

> The journey is the reward.
> —*Tao Proverb*

Physical Activities

Many people find they have more energy when they take part in physical activities such as swimming, walking, yoga, and biking. They find that these types of activities help them keep strong and make them feel good. A bit of exercise everyday:

- improves your chances of feeling better
- keeps your muscles toned
- speeds your healing
- controls stress
- helps free your mind of bad thoughts

Even if you have never done physical activities before, you can start now. Choose something you think you'd like to do, and get your doctor's okay to try it. You can do some exercises even if you have to stay in bed.

Start slowly, doing an activity for just 5 or 10 minutes a day. When you feel strong enough, you can slowly increase this time to 30 minutes or more. Let your doctors and nurses know if you have pain when you do this activity.

Working

People with cancer often want to get back to work. Their jobs not only give them an income but also a sense of routine. Work helps people feel good about themselves.

Before you go back to work, talk with your doctor as well as your boss. Make sure you are well enough to do your job. You may need to work fewer hours or do your job in a different way. Some people feel well enough to work while they are having chemo or radiation treatment. Others need to wait until their treatments are over.

Talking With Your Boss and Co-Workers

"I was nervous about going back to work. A big issue was what to tell my supervisor and co-workers. I knew that they would be supportive, but I was afraid that they would think I was no longer able to do as good a job as I used to."

You might find that your boss and co-workers treat you differently than they did before you had cancer. They may say nothing because they don't know what to say and don't want to hurt your feelings. Or they may not know if you want to talk about your cancer or would rather just focus on work.

If you can, use humor or make a joke. Humor can help break the ice and make people feel more at ease. Let your boss and co-workers know if, and when, you want to talk about your cancer. You may find that it is easier than you thought it would be.

Your Legal Rights

Some people with cancer face roadblocks when they try to go back to work or get a new job. Even those who had cancer many years ago may still have trouble. Employers may not treat them fairly because they believe myths that aren't true. They may believe cancer can be spread from person to person or people with cancer take too many sick days. Some employers also think that people with cancer are poor insurance risks.

It is against the law to discriminate against (treat unfairly) workers who have disabilities such as cancer. These national laws protect your rights as a worker:

- The Federal Rehabilitation Act of 1973
- The Americans With Disabilities Act of 1990

Most states also have laws that protect the rights of people with cancer. You can take legal action (sue) if you think that you are not being hired for a job because of your cancer. Here are some ways to learn more about your legal rights:

- Talk with your social worker and ask about laws in your state. Your social worker can also give you the name of the state agency that protects your rights as an employee.
- Contact your state's Department of Labor or Office of Civil Rights.

- Contact your state Representative or Senator. You can find out who represents your district and how to contact this person by looking on the Internet or at a library.

- Visit the Web site for the National Cancer Institute's State Cancer Legislative Database Program at **http://www.scld-nci.net/**

You may also want to learn about the benefits you can get as a person with cancer. One is the Family and Medical Leave Act. This law allows most workers to take up to 12 weeks of unpaid time to deal with certain family and medical problems. To learn more, speak with the Human Resource office where you work. You can also contact the U.S. Department of Labor at (202) 693-0066 or **http://www.dol.gov/**.

Some people can't return to their jobs because of their cancer. For instance, you may no longer be able to lift heavy boxes if that task is a part of your job. If you can't do the work you did before, contact your state Rehabilitation Program. Ask about training programs that teach you the skills you need for other kinds of work. To learn more, look under the state government section in the blue pages of your phone book.

Thinking About the Future

You may find it helpful to look beyond your treatment and think about what you want to do when you feel well again. Many people find it helpful to set goals. Setting goals gives them something to think about and work toward. Goals can also help people focus on what they want to achieve next week, next year, and into the future. As one man with cancer said,

"I decided I would travel to Europe when my therapy was over. I used treatment time to research the countries I wanted to visit and read first-person accounts written by other travelers. I bought a new camera and figured out how to use it. I even brushed up on my French!"

Goals can also help you get you through hard times. In fact, many cancer patients have done much better than their doctor expected because they wanted to go to a wedding or meet their new grandchild.

It is wise for people with cancer to "put their house in order." Think about making a will and talk about end-of-life choices with your loved ones. You may also want to put your photos into albums, write down your family history, and sort through some of the things you own.

Putting your house in order is not the same as giving up. In fact, it is a way that people with cancer can live each day to the fullest and think about the future. These things make sense for everyone, sick or well.

> If you wait for tomorrow, tomorrow comes.
> If you don't wait for tomorrow, tomorrow comes.
> —*Senegalese Proverb*

Advance Directives

Advance directives are legal papers that allow you to decide ahead of time how you want to be treated when you are dying. They help your loved ones and doctors know what to do if, and when, you can't tell them yourself.

People with cancer face a lot of choices about the future. It's hard to talk about the end of your life. But when you do, you can have peace of mind. You will know you cared enough to make hard choices for yourself, instead of leaving them for your loved ones and health care providers.

Advance directives include:

- A **will** to divide your money and things you own among your heirs

- A **living will** to let people know what kind of medical care you want if you are close to death

- A **durable power of attorney** to appoint a person (a "health care proxy") to make medical decisions for you when you can't make them yourself

- A **trust** to give your money or things you own to someone else

For more information, contact the Cancer Information Service at 1-800-4-CANCER (1-800-422-6237), by TTY (for deaf and hard of hearing callers) at 1-800-332-8615, or through the Internet at **http://cancer.gov**. Click on the Live Help button to send a message.

Once you finish treatment, you may expect life to return to the way it was before cancer. In truth, it can take a while for life to settle down. This can be a hard time. While you adjust to life after treatment, you may find it helpful to read *Facing Forward: Life After Cancer Treatment.* To order a free copy, contact the Cancer Information Service or view it online at **http://cancer.gov**.

Summing Up: Living Each Day

Living with cancer means not only looking at death but also how to live the rest of your life—whether it is long or short. Take care of daily duties and do things that are fun. Both are needed for a full life.

Many people who have cancer feel that living each day to the fullest means:

- staying involved in the duties and pleasures of daily life
- returning to work if possible
- making plans for the future

Resources for Learning More

You may want more information for yourself, your family, and your doctor. These services from the National Cancer Institute (NCI) may help you.

Phone

Cancer Information Service (CIS)
Provides accurate, up-to-date information on cancer to patients and their families, health professionals, and the general public. Information specialists translate the latest scientific information into understandable language and respond in English, Spanish, or on TTY equipment.

Toll-free: 1-800-4-CANCER (1-800-422-6237)
TTY (for deaf and hard of hearing callers): 1-800-332-8615

Internet

http://cancer.gov
NCI's Web site contains comprehensive information about coping with cancer, cancer causes and prevention, screening and diagnosis, treatment and survivorship; clinical trials; statistics; funding, training, and employment opportunities; and the Institute and its programs.

...to find other cancer groups....

Facing Forward: Life After Cancer Treatment
This booklet contains information about many groups that provide services to people with cancer. To obtain a copy, contact the Cancer Information Service or view it online at **http://cancer.gov**.